HEY FELLA, TIME TO LOSE WEIGHT

Cultivating Awareness to Transform Your Body

Sage W. Vesper

Copyright © 2024 by Sage W. Vesper

All rights reserved. Reproduction, distribution, or transmission of any kind, including photocopying, recording, or any other electronic or mechanical methods, is strictly prohibited without the prior written permission of the publisher, except in the case of brief quotations embodied in critical reviews and certain other noncommercial uses permitted by copyright law.

Published by Hannah Digital Media

TABLE OF CONTENT

INTRODUCTION

Hey Fella, Time to Lose Weight

So, you've decided it's time to shed a few pounds and get in shape? That's awesome! I know the idea of losing weight can be daunting, but trust me, it doesn't have to be. This book is your new best friend on this journey. We're going to make it fun, practical, and absolutely achievable. Forget about the fads and unrealistic expectations—this is about real, sustainable change that fits into your life.

Why This Book is Your New Best Friend

You're not just buying a book; you're investing in a healthier, happier you. Here's why you shouldn't waste another second thinking about it:

Real Talk: No fluff, just straightforward advice and strategies that work.

Practical Tips: Easy-to-implement tips that fit into your daily routine.

Motivation Boost: Stay inspired with real-life success stories and encouraging words.

Structured Plan: A step-by-step guide that makes the process simple and manageable.

Results-Oriented: Focused on helping you see and feel the results, not just read about them.

What to Expect on This Journey

Embarking on a weight loss journey can feel overwhelming, but with this book, you'll have a clear path to follow. Here's what you can expect:

Mindset Shifts: We'll start by setting realistic goals and building a positive attitude. You'll learn how to overcome common obstacles and set yourself up for success.

Nutrition Basics: You'll get a solid understanding of calories, macros, and how to fuel your body properly. Plus, you'll find simple meal plans and smart snacking tips.

Exercise Plans: We'll explore different types of workouts and help you find the ones that fit your lifestyle. Whether you prefer the gym or home workouts, there's something for everyone.

Lifestyle Tweaks: Small changes can lead to big results. We'll cover the importance of sleep, stress management techniques, and how to build healthy habits that stick.

Staying Motivated: Learn how to track your progress, celebrate milestones, and stay inspired with stories of people who've been where you are and achieved their goals.

Troubleshooting and Adjusting: Not everything goes as planned. We'll help you handle plateaus, setbacks, and make necessary adjustments to keep moving forward.

By the end of this book, you'll have the knowledge, tools, and confidence to transform your life. It's time to lose weight and gain a healthier, happier you. Let's get started!

CHAPTER 1

Mindset Matters: Preparing for Success

In today's fast-paced, digitally connected world, cultivating the right mindset is crucial for successful weight loss. The journey isn't just about physical transformation but also mental resilience. Here, we'll explore how setting realistic goals, building a positive attitude, and overcoming common obstacles can help you achieve lasting success, with a focus on current trends and examples.

1.1 Setting Realistic Goals

The influence of social media and quick-fix diets can make setting realistic goals challenging. Here's how to stay grounded amidst these trends:

Avoiding Comparison Traps: Platforms like Instagram and TikTok are filled with dramatic before-and-after photos. While these can be inspiring, they can also set unrealistic expectations. Remember, many of these images are filtered and don't show the full journey. Focus on your personal progress and set goals that are tailored to your body and lifestyle. **Example:** Instead of aiming to look like a fitness influencer, set a goal to lose 1-2 pounds per week. This is a sustainable rate of weight loss recommended by health professionals.

Micro-Goals and Celebrations: Breaking down your larger goal into smaller, actionable steps can make the process less overwhelming and more rewarding. **Example:** If your goal is to lose 30 pounds, start with a goal to lose 5 pounds in the first month. Celebrate this achievement with a non-food reward, like a new workout outfit or a fun activity.

Holistic Health Focus: Shift your focus from purely weight loss to overall health improvements, such as better sleep, increased energy, and improved mood. **Example:** Set goals like "I want to improve my sleep quality by getting 7-8 hours of sleep per night" or "I want to increase my daily steps to 10,000."

1.2 Building a Positive Attitude

In an era where mental health is finally receiving the attention it deserves, building a positive attitude is crucial for sustaining your weight loss journey:

Mental Health Awareness: Understand the significant impact of mental health on weight loss. Engaging in activities such as mindfulness, meditation, and therapy can be beneficial in controlling stress and emotional eating. **Example:** Use mindfulness apps like Headspace or Calm to incorporate short meditation sessions into your daily routine. This can help you stay focused and reduce stress.

Digital Detox: Reducing screen time, especially on social media, can prevent negative comparisons and information overload. **Example:** Designate specific times of the day for checking social media and turn off notifications during meals and workouts to stay present and engaged.

Positive Affirmations and Journaling: Reinforce your self-worth and motivation with positive affirmations and by keeping a journal of your progress and feelings. **Example:** Start your day by writing down three positive affirmations, such as "I am capable," "I am committed to my health," and "I am making progress." Reflect on your daily achievements in a journal each night.

1.3 Overcoming Common Obstacles

Modern life is full of challenges that can derail your weight loss efforts. Here's how to navigate some of today's most common obstacles:

Work-from-Home Challenges: With more people working from home, maintaining a healthy routine can be difficult. Create clear boundaries and schedule regular breaks for physical activity. **Example:** Set a timer to remind yourself to stand up and stretch every hour. Incorporate a short walk or quick workout during lunch breaks to stay active.

Pandemic Fatigue and Stress: The lingering effects of the pandemic have led to increased stress and disrupted routines. Be compassionate with yourself and focus on what you can control. **Example:** Establish a consistent daily routine that includes time for self-care, exercise, and healthy meals. Practice stress-relief techniques like deep breathing exercises or yoga.

Information Overload: The internet is full of conflicting advice on weight loss. Make sure to rely on trustworthy sources and consult with a professional for advice. **Example:** Follow advice from trusted health organizations like the CDC or WHO, and consider consulting a registered dietitian or certified personal trainer for personalized support.

Trending Tools and Resources

Leveraging the latest tools and resources can also support your journey:

Fitness Apps: Apps like MyFitnessPal, Fitbit, and Noom offer personalized plans, track your progress, and provide a community for support. **Example:** Use MyFitnessPal to log your meals and track your calorie intake. Join Fitbit challenges to stay motivated by friendly competition with friends and family.

Virtual Workouts: Online platforms like Peloton, Beachbody, and YouTube offer a variety of workouts that you can do from home, catering to different fitness levels and preferences. **Example:** Subscribe to a YouTube channel that offers free, high-quality workouts that fit your interests, whether it's yoga, strength training, or dance.

Telehealth Services: Access to virtual consultations with nutritionists and therapists has made it easier to get professional guidance without leaving your home. **Example:** Schedule regular check-ins with a registered dietitian through telehealth platforms to receive personalized advice and accountability.

By setting realistic goals, maintaining a positive attitude, and being prepared to tackle common obstacles, you'll be well-equipped to navigate the modern challenges of weight loss. Just keep moving forward and you'll start seeing the progress you want. Progress matters more than perfection.

CHAPTER 2

Nutrition: Fueling Your Body Right

Nutrition is the cornerstone of any weight loss journey. With the abundance of diet trends and conflicting information, it can be challenging to know what really works. This chapter focuses on understanding calories and macros, providing simple meal plans and recipes, and offering smart snacking tips to help you fuel your body right.

2.1 Understanding Calories and Macros

In today's world of keto, intermittent fasting, and other trending diets, understanding the basics of calories and macronutrients (macros) is more important than ever:

Calories In vs. Calories Out: The fundamental principle of weight loss is creating a calorie deficit, meaning you consume fewer calories than you burn. However, the quality of those calories also matters. **Example:** Eating 1,500 calories of nutrient-dense foods like vegetables, lean proteins, and whole grains will support your health better than 1,500 calories of junk food.

Macronutrients: Macros are the nutrients that provide energy: carbohydrates, proteins, and fats. Every one has an important part to play in your diet. **Example:** A balanced macro distribution might look like 40% carbohydrates, 30% protein, and 30% fat. Adjust these ratios based on your personal needs and goals.

Trending Insight: High-protein diets are popular for their role in muscle building and satiety. Consider incorporating more lean proteins like chicken, fish, tofu, and legumes into your meals.

2.2 Simple Meal Plans and Recipes

With busy lifestyles and the constant temptation of convenience foods, simple meal plans and easy recipes are essential for staying on track:

Batch Cooking: Preparing meals in advance can save time and ensure you have healthy options available throughout the week. **Example:** Spend a couple of hours on Sunday cooking large batches of quinoa, grilled chicken, and roasted vegetables. Store them in individual containers for quick, nutritious meals.

One-Pan Dinners: Simplify your cooking routine with one-pan meals that minimize cleanup and maximize flavor. **Example:** Try a sheet pan dinner with salmon, asparagus, and sweet potatoes. Season with olive oil, lemon, and your favorite herbs, then bake at 400°F for 20-25 minutes.

Trending Recipe: Overnight oats have become a breakfast favorite for their convenience and versatility. Combine rolled oats, Greek yogurt, almond milk, chia seeds, and a bit of honey. Refrigerate overnight and top with fresh fruit in the morning.

2.3 Smart Snacking Tips

Snacking can be a major pitfall if not managed correctly. Here are some smart snacking strategies that align with current trends:

Mindful Snacking: Avoid mindless eating by paying attention to your snacks. Choose nutrient-dense options that satisfy hunger and provide energy. **Example:** Instead of reaching for a bag of chips, opt for a small handful of nuts and a piece of fruit.

Protein-Packed Snacks: High-protein snacks can help keep you full between meals and support muscle maintenance. **Example:** Snack on Greek yogurt with a sprinkle of granola, or keep hard-boiled eggs handy for a quick protein boost.

Trending Snack: Energy balls are a popular, easy-to-make snack. Combine rolled oats, nut butter, honey, and mix-ins like chocolate chips or dried fruit. Shape into balls and chill in the fridge for a convenient snack on the run.

Leveraging Technology

Use technology to help you stay on track with your nutrition:

Nutrition Apps: Apps like MyFitnessPal and Lose It! can help you track your calorie intake and macro distribution, making it easier to stay within your goals. **Example:** Use MyFitnessPal to scan barcodes and log your meals. The app provides detailed nutritional information and tracks your progress over time.

Meal Delivery Services: If cooking isn't your thing or you're pressed for time, consider using meal delivery services that focus on healthy, balanced meals. **Example:** Services like HelloFresh and Blue Apron offer pre-portioned ingredients and simple recipes that make cooking at home convenient and nutritious.

By understanding calories and macros, following simple meal plans and recipes, and adopting smart snacking habits, you can fuel your body right and stay on track with your weight loss goals. Embrace these strategies and leverage the latest tools to make nutrition a manageable and enjoyable part of your daily routine.

CHAPTER 3

Exercise: Moving Toward a Healthier You

Exercise is a vital component of any weight loss journey, contributing not only to calorie burning but also to overall health and well-being. This chapter explores trends and offers examples on finding the right workout, incorporating physical activity into your day, and deciding between home and gym workouts.

3.1 Finding the Right Workout for You

In a fitness landscape filled with diverse options, finding the right workout that suits your preferences and lifestyle is key:

Personalized Fitness Plans: Tailoring your workout routine to your fitness level, goals, and interests can enhance motivation and enjoyment. **Example:** If you enjoy group activities, consider joining a local fitness class or trying a virtual workout community like Peloton or Fitness Blender.

Functional Training: Functional fitness, which focuses on movements that mimic everyday activities, has gained popularity for its practical benefits.

Trending Insight: Incorporating exercises like squats, lunges, and planks not only strengthens muscles but also improves balance and flexibility, supporting overall fitness and reducing injury risk.

Hybrid Workouts: Combining different types of exercises—such as cardio, strength training, and flexibility work—into one session can maximize workout efficiency and effectiveness. **Example:** Try a HIIT (High-Intensity Interval Training) workout that alternates between bursts of intense activity and short rest periods to burn calories and improve cardiovascular health.

3.2 Incorporating Physical Activity into Your Day

In today's sedentary lifestyles, finding ways to incorporate movement throughout the day is crucial for overall health:

Active Commuting: Walking or biking to work, or getting off public transport a stop early, can add valuable physical activity to your day. **Example:** If feasible, consider incorporating a morning walk or bike ride into your commute routine to jump-start your day with movement.

Desk Exercises: Short bursts of exercise at your desk, such as stretching, leg lifts, or desk yoga, can improve circulation and reduce stiffness.

Trending Insight: Apps like DeskCycle and Cubii offer under-desk exercise equipment designed to keep you active while working.

Fitness Trackers: Wearable technology, such as fitness trackers and smart watches, can motivate you to meet daily activity goals by monitoring steps, heart rate, and even sleep patterns. **Example:** Set reminders to move throughout the day based on your activity level tracked by your fitness tracker, encouraging regular breaks and movement.

3.3 Home Workouts vs. Gym Workouts

The debate between home and gym workouts has intensified, influenced by convenience, cost-effectiveness, and personal preferences:

Home Workouts: The convenience of exercising at home has surged with the rise of virtual fitness platforms and on-demand workout videos. **Example:** Follow online fitness channels like Yoga with Adriene or Fitness Blender for guided workouts that cater to various fitness levels and goals.

Gym Workouts: Access to specialized equipment and the motivational environment of a gym can enhance workout intensity and variety.

Trending Insight: Boutique fitness studios, offering specialized classes like spin, barre, or boxing, provide a unique workout experience with professional guidance and community support.

Hybrid Approach: Many fitness enthusiasts adopt a hybrid approach, combining home workouts for convenience with occasional gym visits for equipment-based training or social interaction. **Example:** Use a fitness app to design your home workout routine and attend a weekly group fitness class at your local gym for additional motivation and variety.

Leveraging Virtual Fitness

Virtual fitness has revolutionized how people access workouts, offering flexibility and variety:

Live Streaming Classes: Participate in real-time workouts led by professional trainers from the comfort of your home. **Example:** Platforms like Zoom and Instagram Live offer live fitness classes ranging from yoga and dance to strength training and cardio.

On-Demand Workouts: Access pre-recorded workout videos that you can stream anytime, anywhere, allowing you to customize your fitness schedule. **Example:** Subscribe to platforms like Beachbody On Demand or Les Mills On Demand for a wide range of workout programs, from beginner to advanced levels.

By exploring different workout options, integrating physical activity into your daily routine, and deciding on the best setting—whether home or gym—you can create a fitness regimen that supports your weight loss goals and enhances your overall well-being. Embrace the trends that resonate with you and adapt your approach over time to stay motivated and engaged in your fitness journey.

CHAPTER 4

Lifestyle Changes: Small Tweaks, Big Results

Lifestyle adjustments can make a real difference in your efforts to lose weight. Small, consistent tweaks can lead to substantial results over time. This chapter explores trends and examples on the crucial roles of sleep, stress management, and building healthy habits.

4.1 Sleep and Its Role in Weight Loss

Sleep is often an overlooked component of weight loss, but its importance cannot be overstated:

Quality Over Quantity: While getting enough sleep is important, the quality of sleep also matters. Deep, restorative sleep is crucial for hormone regulation and overall health.

Example: Aim for 7-9 hours of high-quality sleep per night by creating a relaxing bedtime routine and ensuring your sleep environment is comfortable and free from distractions.

Sleep and Metabolism: Poor sleep can disrupt your metabolism and increase hunger hormones like ghrelin while decreasing satiety hormones like leptin.

Trending Insight: Incorporate practices such as limiting caffeine intake, reducing screen time before bed, and maintaining a consistent sleep schedule to improve sleep quality and support weight loss.

Wearable Sleep Trackers: Technology can help monitor and improve your sleep patterns. Devices like Fitbit and the Oura Ring track sleep stages and offer insights for better sleep habits. **Example:** Use a sleep tracker to analyze your sleep data and identify patterns or behaviors that might be affecting your sleep quality, then adjust your routine accordingly.

4.2 Stress Management Techniques

Weight loss goals can be derailed by chronic stress, leading to emotional eating and hormonal imbalances. Managing stress effectively is key to maintaining a healthy lifestyle:

Mindfulness and Meditation: Practices like mindfulness and meditation can reduce stress and promote emotional well-being. **Example:** Use apps like Headspace or Calm for guided meditation sessions that fit into your daily routine, helping you to manage stress and stay focused on your goals.

Physical Activity: Exercise is a natural stress reliever. Activities such as yoga, tai chi, and walking can help lower stress levels and improve mood.

Trending Insight: Incorporate low-intensity, stress-reducing exercises into your fitness regimen. Yoga with Adriene on YouTube offers a variety of yoga practices specifically designed for relaxation and stress relief.

Getting involved in creative activities such as painting, writing, or playing music can be really therapeutic and help lower stress levels. **Example:** Dedicate time each week to a hobby you enjoy. This not only reduces stress but also provides a productive way to unwind.

4.3 Building Healthy Habits

Creating and maintaining healthy habits is essential for long-term success. Small changes can lead to big results when integrated consistently into your daily routine:

Habit Stacking: This technique involves adding a new habit to an existing one to make it easier to incorporate into your routine. **Example:** If you already have a morning coffee ritual, use this time to also take a multivitamin or do a quick 5-minute stretch. This links the new habit to an established one, making it easier to remember and stick to.

Accountability Partners: Having someone to share your goals with can provide motivation and accountability.

Trending Insight: Join online communities or find a workout buddy to share your progress and challenges. Platforms like MyFitnessPal and Strava have built-in social features for this purpose.

Digital Habit Trackers: Apps like HabitBull or Streaks help you track and reinforce new habits by providing reminders and visualizing your progress. **Example:** Use a habit tracker to set and monitor daily goals, such as drinking eight glasses of water, taking a 10-minute walk, or practicing gratitude journaling.

Embracing a Holistic Approach

A holistic approach to lifestyle changes involves addressing multiple aspects of health and well-being:

Balanced Nutrition: Focus on whole, nutrient-dense foods that fuel your body and support overall health. **Example:** Plan your meals to include a variety of vegetables, lean proteins, healthy fats, and whole grains. Apps like Yummly can provide healthy recipe ideas tailored to your preferences.

Mind-Body Connection: Practices that integrate the mind and body can enhance overall well-being and support weight loss.

Trending Insight: Mind-body practices like Qigong or Pilates emphasize the connection between physical movement and mental focus, promoting holistic health.

Sustainable Changes: Aim for changes that you can maintain long-term, rather than quick fixes that are difficult to sustain. **Example:** Instead of drastically cutting out all carbs, focus on replacing refined grains with whole grains and increasing your intake of vegetables and lean proteins.

By prioritizing quality sleep, managing stress effectively, and building sustainable healthy habits, you can make small tweaks that lead to big results. Embrace these lifestyle changes and use the latest trends and tools to support your journey toward a healthier, happier you.

CHAPTER 5

Staying Motivated: Keeping the Momentum Going

Embarking on a weight loss journey is one thing; staying motivated and keeping the momentum going is another. It's common to experience fluctuations in motivation, but by tracking your progress, celebrating milestones, and staying inspired with success stories, you can sustain your enthusiasm and achieve your goals. This chapter explores these strategies with trends and examples to help you maintain your drive.

5.1 Tracking Your Progress

Keeping track of your progress can really help you stay motivated. It provides tangible evidence of your efforts and helps you make necessary adjustments along the way. Check out these latest trends and examples:

Wearable Technology: Fitness trackers like Fitbit, Apple Watch, and Garmin have become incredibly popular for their ability to monitor various health metrics, including steps taken, calories burned, heart rate, and even sleep quality.

Example: Using a Fitbit, you can set a daily step goal and monitor your progress throughout the day. The app provides detailed insights into your activity levels and can help you identify patterns and areas for improvement.

Digital Health Apps: Apps like MyFitnessPal, Lose It!, and Noom allow you to log your food intake, track calories, and monitor your exercise routines. These apps often include community features where you can share your progress and get support from others.

Example: MyFitnessPal lets you scan food barcodes to quickly log your meals, making it easier to keep track of your nutritional intake. It also provides a visual representation of your calorie intake versus your calorie burn, helping you stay on track.

Progress Photos: Taking regular photos can provide a visual record of your transformation, offering a powerful reminder of how far you've come. **Example:** Take a photo once a month in the same outfit and from the same angle. Compare these photos over time to see your physical changes, which can be incredibly motivating.

Body Measurements: In addition to tracking weight, measuring different parts of your body can provide a more comprehensive picture of your progress. This can include measurements of your waist, hips, thighs, and arms. **Example:** Use a tape measure to record your measurements every two weeks. Sometimes, you may lose inches even if the scale doesn't move, indicating fat loss and muscle gain.

5.2 Celebrating Milestones

Celebrating milestones along your weight loss journey is essential for maintaining motivation. Recognizing and rewarding your achievements keeps you focused and provides a positive reinforcement mechanism. Here's how to celebrate effectively:

Set Mini-Goals: Breaking down your larger weight loss goal into smaller, manageable milestones can make the journey feel less daunting and more achievable.

Example: If your goal is to lose 50 pounds, set mini-goals for every 10 pounds lost. Celebrate each achievement with a non-food reward, like a new workout outfit or a massage.

Reward System: Develop a reward system that aligns with your interests and keeps you motivated to reach your goals. **Example:** Create a list of rewards for different milestones. This could include a weekend getaway for hitting the halfway mark or a new gadget for reaching your ultimate goal.

Social Celebrations: Share your milestones with friends and family. Their encouragement and recognition can provide an additional motivational boost. **Example:** Host a virtual or in-person celebration with your support network each time you hit a major milestone. This could be a small gathering or a fun activity that you enjoy.

Reflect and Reassess: Take time to reflect on your journey and reassess your goals periodically. Utilizing this can keep you focused and ready to make any adjustments if needed. **Example:** Keep a journal where you write about your progress, challenges, and successes. Use this as an opportunity to celebrate your achievements and plan your next steps.

5.3 Staying Inspired with Success Stories

Hearing about others' successes can provide a powerful source of motivation. Success stories remind us that achieving our goals is possible and offer practical tips and inspiration. Here's how to leverage success stories effectively:

Online Communities: Joining online weight loss communities like Reddit's r/loseit or forums on websites like Weight Watchers can provide access to countless success stories and a supportive network. **Example:** Participate in discussions, share your journey, and read about others' experiences. These stories can provide tips, encouragement, and a sense of camaraderie.

Social Media Influencers: Follow influencers and bloggers who share their weight loss journeys on platforms like Instagram, YouTube, or TikTok. Many of them offer honest accounts of their struggles and successes, along with practical advice. **Example:** Follow an influencer who has a similar body type or goals as you. Seeing their progress and tips can be incredibly motivating and relatable.

Weight Loss Books and Documentaries: Reading books or watching documentaries about weight loss can offer in-depth insights and inspiration. **Example:** Watch documentaries like "Fat, Sick & Nearly Dead" or read books like "The

Obesity Code" by Dr. Jason Fung. These resources can provide valuable knowledge and motivational stories.

Personal Connections: Talk to friends, family, or colleagues who have successfully lost weight. Personal connections can offer encouragement and firsthand advice.

Example: If you know someone who has achieved significant weight loss, ask them to share their journey with you. Their insights and encouragement can be incredibly motivating.

Combining Strategies for Long-Term Success

Combining these strategies—tracking progress, celebrating milestones, and staying inspired with success stories—can create a comprehensive approach to maintaining motivation throughout your weight loss journey.

Integrated Approach: Use a fitness tracker to monitor your daily activity and an app to log your meals. Take progress photos and body measurements regularly. Celebrate each milestone with a planned reward and share your achievements with your support network. **Example:** Set up a weekly routine where you review your progress, adjust your goals if needed, and plan a small celebration for your next milestone. This integrated approach keeps you engaged and motivated.

Support System: Build a support system that includes friends, family, online communities, and perhaps a mentor or coach who can provide guidance and encouragement. **Example:** Join a local fitness class or online challenge group where members share their progress and support each other. Having a community can make the journey feel less isolating and more collaborative.

Continuous Learning: Stay informed about new trends, techniques, and success stories in the weight loss world. This can keep your routine fresh and prevent boredom. **Example:** Subscribe to fitness and health blogs, podcasts, or YouTube channels that regularly share new information and inspiring stories. Implement new strategies that resonate with you.

Mindfulness and Self-Compassion: Practice mindfulness and self-compassion to maintain a positive mindset, even when facing setbacks. **Example:** Incorporate mindfulness practices like meditation or yoga into your routine. Always be kind to yourself and accept that setbacks are a regular part of the journey.

By adopting these strategies and staying proactive in your approach, you can keep your motivation high and maintain the momentum needed to achieve your weight loss goals. Remember, the journey is as important as the destination, and staying motivated is the key to long-term success.

CHAPTER 6

Troubleshooting: When Things Don't Go as Planned

Weight loss journeys are rarely linear. You might encounter plateaus, setbacks, and the need to adjust your plan along the way. Understanding how to troubleshoot these challenges effectively can keep you on track and help you achieve your goals. This chapter addresses dealing with plateaus, handling setbacks, and adjusting your plan for continued success, using current trends and practical examples.

6.1 Dealing with Plateaus

It's common to experience a weight loss plateau, and it can be quite frustrating. They occur when your weight loss stalls despite maintaining your diet and exercise routines. Here's how to break through these plateaus:

.Reassessing and adjusting your caloric intake can help restart weight loss. **Example:** Use a calorie calculator to determine your new daily caloric needs based on your current weight and activity level. Apps like MyFitnessPal can help you track your adjusted intake.

Increase Exercise Intensity: Your body adapts to your workout routine over time. Increasing the intensity or changing your exercise regimen can challenge your body and break the plateau.

Trending Insight: High-Intensity Interval Training (HIIT) is popular for its effectiveness in burning fat and boosting metabolism. Try incorporating HIIT workouts into your routine to increase calorie burn. **Example:** Replace one of your regular cardio sessions with a 20-minute HIIT workout, alternating between 30 seconds of intense exercise and 30 seconds of rest.

Vary Your Workouts: Adding variety to your workouts can prevent boredom and keep your body guessing. **Example:** If you usually run, try swimming or cycling. Join a new fitness class like Zumba, kickboxing, or Pilates to work different muscle groups and maintain interest.

Monitor Macronutrient Ratios: Sometimes, adjusting the balance of proteins, fats, and carbohydrates in your diet can help overcome a plateau.

Trending Insight: The ketogenic diet, which emphasizes high fat, moderate protein, and low carbohydrate intake, has been shown to break plateaus for some people. **Example:** Consult with a nutritionist to see if adjusting your macronutrient ratios could benefit you. Test different ratios to see which one is most effective for your body.

6.2 Handling Setbacks

Facing obstacles is a natural part of every weight loss process.How you handle them can make all the difference in achieving long-term success. Here's how to manage and bounce back from setbacks:

Practice Self-Compassion: Being kind to yourself during setbacks can reduce stress and prevent a negative spiral.

Trending Insight: Self-compassion techniques, including positive self-talk and mindfulness, are increasingly recognized for their role in maintaining mental health and resilience. **Example:** When you experience a setback, remind yourself that it's a normal part of the process. Engage in mindfulness meditation to remain rooted and alleviate stress.

Analyze the Cause: Understanding what led to the setback can help you avoid similar situations in the future. **Example:** If you find yourself overeating during stressful periods, identify the triggers and develop healthier coping mechanisms, such as going for a walk, journaling, or practicing deep breathing exercises.

Create an Action Plan: Develop a clear plan to get back on track after a setback. This includes setting new, realistic goals and outlining specific steps to achieve them. **Example:** If you've fallen off your workout routine, set a small goal to exercise for 10 minutes each day for the next week. Gradually increase the duration as you regain your momentum.

Seek Support: Sharing your struggles with friends, family, or a support group can provide encouragement and accountability.

Trending Insight: Online communities and social media groups focused on weight loss can offer a supportive environment for sharing experiences and receiving advice.
Example: Join a Facebook group dedicated to weight loss where members share their challenges and successes. Engage with the community to stay motivated and supported.

6.3 Adjusting Your Plan for Continued Success

Flexibility is key to maintaining progress. As you advance in your weight loss journey, you may need to adjust your plan to reflect changes in your body, lifestyle, and goals. Here's how to adapt your plan for continued success:

Reevaluate Your Goals: Regularly assess your short-term and long-term goals to ensure they remain realistic and achievable. **Example:** If your initial goal was to lose 50 pounds, break it down into smaller milestones. Once you reach each milestone, set a new goal to keep you motivated.

Update Your Exercise Routine: Changing your workout routine can prevent plateaus and keep you engaged.

Trending Insight: Functional fitness training, which focuses on exercises that improve daily activities, is gaining popularity. It's important to mix in functional exercises like squats, lunges, and push-ups when you work out. **Example:** Every few months, switch up your exercise regimen. If you've been focusing on cardio, add strength training to your routine. Consider working with a personal trainer to develop a varied workout plan.

Adjust Your Diet: As you progress, your nutritional needs may change. Make sure to consistently check your diet and make any needed changes. **Example:** If you've been following a low-carb diet, consider gradually reintroducing healthy carbs like quinoa, sweet potatoes, and fruits. Watch how your body responds and adapt as necessary.

Incorporate New Technologies: Utilize the latest fitness and nutrition technologies to stay on track and motivated. **Trending Insight:** Virtual fitness classes and telehealth consultations with nutritionists are becoming more accessible and can provide personalized guidance and support. **Example:** Sign up for a virtual fitness class subscription service like Peloton or Beachbody On Demand. Schedule regular telehealth consultations with a nutritionist to ensure your diet aligns with your goals.

Practical Examples and Success Stories

To illustrate these strategies, here are some practical examples and success stories:

Case Study 1: Breaking Through a Plateau

Sarah's Story: Sarah hit a plateau after losing 20 pounds. Despite maintaining her diet and exercise routine, her weight wouldn't budge. She decided to reassess her caloric needs and found that she needed to reduce her intake by 200 calories per day. She also added HIIT workouts to her routine and saw immediate progress. Within a month, she broke through her plateau and continued losing weight.

Case Study 2: Overcoming Setbacks

John's Story: John faced a major setback when he injured his knee, preventing him from continuing his usual running routine. He felt discouraged and gained back some weight. After practicing self-compassion and seeking support from an online community, he developed a new action plan. He started swimming and doing upper-body strength training while his knee healed. This kept him active and motivated, and he was able to get back on track.

Emma's Story: Emma reached her initial goal of losing 30 pounds but wanted to continue improving her fitness. She reevaluated her goals and decided to focus on building muscle. She updated her exercise routine to include more strength training and adjusted her diet to increase her protein intake. She also joined a virtual fitness community for additional support and motivation. As a result, Emma continued to see progress and felt more confident in her new plan.

Leveraging Professional Guidance

Sometimes, seeking professional help can provide the expertise and accountability needed to overcome challenges and achieve your goals:

Nutritionists and Dietitians: These professionals can offer personalized dietary advice and help you develop a sustainable eating plan.

Trending Insight: Telehealth services have made it easier to access nutritionists and dietitians from the comfort of your home. **Example**: Schedule regular virtual consultations with a dietitian who can help you fine-tune your diet based on your progress and any plateaus or setbacks you encounter.

Personal Trainers: A personal trainer can design a customized workout plan that evolves with your fitness level and goals. **Example:** Work with a personal trainer to create a varied and challenging exercise routine. Stay accountable and adjust as needed by scheduling regular check-ins.

Therapists and Counselors: Emotional and psychological factors play a significant role in weight loss. Therapists can help address issues like emotional eating, stress, and self-esteem. **Example:** Consider seeing a therapist who specializes in weight-related issues. CBT works great for changing negative thought patterns and behaviors.

Troubleshooting is an essential part of any weight loss journey. By learning how to deal with plateaus, handle setbacks, and adjust your plan for continued success, you can maintain your momentum and achieve your goals. Stay informed about the latest trends, seek professional guidance when needed, and remember to practice self-compassion and resilience. Every challenge is an opportunity to learn and grow, bringing you one step closer to a healthier, happier you.

CHAPTER 7

Maintaining Your New Lifestyle: The Long-Term Plan

Reaching your weight loss goal is a significant achievement, but maintaining that success and integrating it into a sustainable lifestyle is equally important. This chapter will cover the key aspects of maintaining your new lifestyle, including keeping the weight off, continuing healthy habits, and evolving your fitness goals. We'll explore current trends and provide practical examples to help you stay on track for the long term.

7.1 Keeping the Weight Off

Maintaining weight loss requires a commitment to the lifestyle changes that helped you shed the pounds in the first place. Check out these tips to maintain your weight loss:

Regular Monitoring: Consistently tracking your weight and health metrics can help you stay aware of any changes and take action before they become significant setbacks.

Trending Insight: Smart scales, such as those from Withings or Fitbit, sync with apps to track weight, body fat percentage, and muscle mass over time. **Example:** Weigh yourself weekly using a smart scale that logs your data. Review your progress monthly to identify trends and adjust your habits as needed.

Balanced Diet: Maintaining a balanced diet is crucial for long-term weight management. Focus on whole foods and avoid reverting to old eating habits.

Trending Insight: The Mediterranean diet, known for its health benefits, emphasizes fruits, vegetables, whole grains, lean proteins, and healthy fats. **Example:** Plan your meals around the Mediterranean diet principles. Incorporate olive oil, fish, nuts, and plenty of vegetables into your daily meals.

Mindful Eating: Being mindful of what and how you eat can prevent overeating and help you make healthier choices.

Trending Insight: Mindful eating practices, including savoring each bite and eating without distractions, are gaining popularity for their effectiveness in weight management. **Example:** Practice mindful eating by eliminating distractions during meals, chewing slowly, and paying attention to hunger and fullness cues. Apps like Eat Right Now can guide you through mindful eating exercises.

Avoiding Yo-Yo Dieting: Yo-yo dieting can lead to metabolic slowdown and weight regain. Focus on maintaining a consistent, healthy diet instead of cyclical dieting. **Example:** If you notice yourself slipping into old habits, return to the basics of balanced nutrition and portion control. Avoid drastic calorie reductions or fad diets.

7.2 Continuing Healthy Habits

The habits that helped you lose weight are essential for maintaining your new lifestyle. Here's how to ensure they become a permanent part of your routine:

Routine Physical Activity: Regular exercise is vital for maintaining weight loss and overall health. Discover hobbies that bring you joy to help you stay inspired.

Trending Insight: Wearable fitness technology, such as fitness trackers and smartwatches, can help you monitor your activity levels and set fitness goals. **Example:** Use a Fitbit or Apple Watch to set a daily step goal, such as 10,000 steps, and track your progress throughout the day. Participate in fitness challenges with friends or online communities to stay motivated.

Healthy Sleep Patterns: Adequate sleep is crucial for weight maintenance and overall health.

Trending Insight: Sleep tracking devices and apps, like the Oura Ring or Sleep Cycle, can help you monitor your sleep quality and make adjustments for better rest.

Example: Establish a consistent sleep schedule and create a bedtime routine to improve your sleep quality. Use a sleep tracker to identify patterns and make necessary changes.

Dealing with Stress: Long-term stress can cause weight gain and various health problems. Adding stress management strategies to your daily schedule can keep you healthy.

Trending Insight: Mindfulness and meditation apps, such as Calm and Headspace, offer guided sessions to reduce stress and improve mental well-being. **Example:** Dedicate 10 minutes each day to mindfulness meditation using an app like Calm. Practice deep breathing exercises or yoga to manage stress effectively.

Regular Check-Ins: Periodically review your habits, goals, and progress to ensure you're staying on track. **Example:** Set aside time each month to reflect on your journey, assess your current habits, and make any necessary adjustments. eep track of your thoughts and progress by using a journal.

7.3 Evolving Your Fitness Goals

As you maintain your weight loss, your fitness goals may evolve. Setting new goals can keep you motivated and improve your overall fitness level:

Strength Training: Incorporating strength training can help build muscle, boost metabolism, and improve body composition.

Trending Insight: Functional fitness training, which focuses on movements that improve daily life activities, is becoming more popular. **Example:** Join a functional fitness class or incorporate exercises like squats, deadlifts, and kettlebell swings into your routine. Make it a goal to do strength training exercises two to three times weekly.

Endurance Activities: Building endurance can improve cardiovascular health and increase overall fitness. **Example:** Set a goal to participate in a local 5K or 10K race. Use a training plan from apps like Couch to 5K to gradually build your endurance and prepare for the event.

Flexibility and Mobility: Improving flexibility and mobility can enhance performance in other activities and reduce the risk of injury.

Trending Insight: Yoga and Pilates are popular for their benefits in flexibility, strength, and mental well-being. **Example:** Incorporate a weekly yoga or Pilates session into your routine. Follow online classes or use apps like Yoga with Adriene for guided practices.

Skill-Based Goals: Setting goals that focus on learning new skills can keep your fitness routine exciting and engaging. **Example:** Challenge yourself to learn a new sport or activity, such as rock climbing, dancing, or swimming. Take lessons or join a group to stay motivated and improve your skills.

Practical Examples and Success Stories

To illustrate these strategies, here are some practical examples and success stories:

Case Study 1: Maintaining Weight Loss

David's Story: David lost 40 pounds by following a low-carb diet and regular exercise routine. To maintain his weight loss, he adopted the Mediterranean diet, which allowed for more variety while still emphasizing healthy foods. David also used a smart scale to track his weight and body composition, ensuring he stayed on track.

Case Study 2: Continuing Healthy Habits

Lisa's Story: Lisa successfully lost 30 pounds by incorporating daily walks and mindful eating practices. To maintain her new lifestyle, she invested in a Fitbit to monitor her activity levels and joined a local hiking club to keep her exercise routine interesting. Lisa also practiced mindfulness meditation using the Headspace app to manage stress.

Case Study 3: Evolving Fitness Goals

Mark's Story: After losing 50 pounds, Mark wanted to build muscle and improve his overall fitness. He started strength training with a personal trainer and set a goal to participate in a Spartan Race. Mark's trainer helped him develop a functional fitness routine that included exercises to improve his strength, endurance, and mobility. Mark also incorporated weekly yoga sessions to enhance his flexibility and reduce the risk of injury.

Leveraging Professional Guidance

Seeking professional guidance can provide the expertise and support needed to maintain your new lifestyle and achieve evolving fitness goals:

Nutritionists and Dietitians: These professionals can help you develop a sustainable eating plan and adjust it as your needs change. **Example:** Schedule regular consultations with a dietitian to ensure your diet remains balanced and supports your long-term goals.

Personal Trainers: A personal trainer can design a customized workout plan that evolves with your fitness level and goals. **Example:** Work with a personal trainer to create a varied and challenging exercise routine. Having consistent check-ins can help you stay accountable and make the right adjustments when needed.

Therapists and Counselors: Emotional and psychological factors play a significant role in weight maintenance. Therapists can help address issues like emotional eating, stress, and self-esteem. **Example:** Consider seeing a therapist who specializes in weight-related issues. CBT works really well in helping to shift negative thinking and behaviors.

Maintaining your new lifestyle is a continuous journey that requires commitment and adaptability. By focusing on keeping the weight off, continuing healthy habits, and evolving your fitness goals, you can ensure long-term success. Embrace the latest trends and technologies, seek professional guidance when needed, and stay motivated by setting new and exciting goals. Remember, the key to maintaining your new lifestyle is finding a balance that works for you and making it an enjoyable and sustainable part of your everyday life.

CHAPTER 8

Resources: Tools and Support for Your Journey

Embarking on and maintaining a weight loss journey can be challenging, but numerous resources are available to support and guide you. This chapter covers recommended apps and websites, community and support groups, and further reading and learning materials. Leveraging these resources can provide you with the tools and encouragement you need to achieve and maintain your weight loss goals.

8.1 Recommended Apps and Websites

Technology has revolutionized the way we approach weight loss and fitness. Here are some of the top apps and websites that can assist you on your journey:

1. **MyFitnessPal**

Description: MyFitnessPal is a popular app for tracking calories, nutrients, and exercise. The app features an extensive range of food options and syncs with a variety of fitness trackers.

Trending Insight: With over 140 million users, MyFitnessPal offers a comprehensive platform for monitoring your diet and physical activity. **Example:** Use MyFitnessPal to log your daily food intake, set calorie goals, and track your macronutrients. The app provides insights into your eating habits and helps you make healthier choices.

2. Lose It!

Description: Lose It! is another excellent app for tracking food intake and exercise. It offers a barcode scanner for easy logging and a supportive community.

Trending Insight: Lose It! uses advanced algorithms to predict your weight loss progress and suggest personalized plans. **Example:** Scan barcodes of food items to quickly add them to your log. Set weight loss goals and join challenges to stay motivated and accountable.

3. Noom

Description: Noom combines the psychology of weight loss with personalized coaching to help users develop healthier habits.

Trending Insight: Noom emphasizes behavioral changes and cognitive-behavioral techniques to create sustainable weight loss. **Example:** Engage with a personal coach through the Noom app to receive tailored advice and support. Participate in daily lessons and activities that focus on changing your mindset and habits.

4. Fitbit

Description: Fitbit offers a range of wearable devices that track physical activity, heart rate, sleep, and more. The accompanying app provides detailed insights and goal-setting features.

Trending Insight: Fitbit's community features and challenges make it easy to stay motivated by connecting with friends and other users. **Example:** Use a Fitbit device to monitor your steps, active minutes, and sleep quality. Join step challenges with friends to keep each other motivated.

5. Cronometer

Description: Cronometer is a detailed nutrition tracking app that focuses on micronutrient intake. It's ideal for those who want to ensure they're getting all essential vitamins and minerals.

Trending Insight: Cronometer's emphasis on micronutrient tracking sets it apart from other apps that primarily focus on macronutrients. **Example:** Log your meals in Cronometer to see a comprehensive breakdown of your nutrient intake. Use this information to adjust your diet and address any deficiencies.

6. Peloton

Description: Peloton offers live and on-demand fitness classes that you can participate in from home. It includes cycling, running, strength, yoga, and more.

Trending Insight: Peloton's engaging classes and community aspect have made it a leader in the home fitness industry. **Example:** Join a live Peloton cycling class to experience the energy and motivation of a group workout from the comfort of your home. Track your progress and set new fitness goals within the app.

8.2 Community and Support Groups

Support from others can be a crucial component of a successful weight loss journey. Here are some ways to connect with communities and support groups:

1. Facebook Groups

Description: Facebook hosts numerous groups focused on weight loss, fitness, and healthy living. These groups provide a platform to share experiences, ask questions, and receive support.

Trending Insight: The diversity of Facebook groups means you can find a community that aligns with your specific goals and interests. **Example:** Join groups like "Keto for Beginners" or "Weight Watchers Support Group" to connect with others who share your dietary preferences and goals. Participate in discussions and share your progress to stay motivated.

2. Reddit Communities

Description: Reddit has various subreddits dedicated to weight loss, fitness, and healthy living, such as r/loseit, r/fitness, and r/keto.

Trending Insight: Reddit's anonymous nature allows for honest sharing and support without the fear of judgment. **Example:** Post your progress photos on r/progresspics to receive encouragement from the community. Ask for advice on r/loseit if you're facing challenges or need tips to stay on track.

3. Weight Watchers (WW) Connect

Description: Weight Watchers offers a social network within their app called Connect, where members can share their journey, support each other, and celebrate successes.

Trending Insight: WW Connect fosters a sense of community and belonging, making it easier to stay committed to the program.

Example: Share your daily meals, workout routines, and weight loss milestones on WW Connect. Engage with other members by commenting on their posts and offering support.

4. Meetup

Description: Meetup is a platform for finding and joining local groups with similar interests, including fitness and weight loss.

Trending Insight: Meetup's in-person gatherings can provide a more personal and tangible sense of community and accountability. **Example:** Search for fitness or weight loss meetups in your area, such as hiking groups, running clubs, or nutrition workshops. Attend these events to make new friends and stay motivated.

5. Instagram

Description: Instagram can be a source of inspiration and motivation through fitness influencers, dietitians, and everyday individuals sharing their weight loss journeys.

Trending Insight: The visual nature of Instagram allows users to share progress photos, healthy recipes, and workout routines. **Example:** Follow fitness influencers who share workout tips and motivational content. Create your own fitness account to document your journey and connect with others.

8.3 Further Reading and Learning

Websites

Healthline

Description: Healthline offers a wealth of articles on nutrition, fitness, and wellness, written and reviewed by medical professionals.

Trending Insight: Healthline's evidence-based approach ensures that the information is accurate and reliable. **Example:** Visit Healthline to read articles on meal planning, exercise routines, and mental health strategies to support your weight loss journey.

Nerd Fitness

Description: Nerd Fitness provides fitness advice, workout plans, and nutrition tips geared toward beginners and those who may feel intimidated by traditional fitness culture.

Trending Insight: Nerd Fitness's community-oriented approach helps users feel supported and motivated. **Example:** Follow Nerd Fitness's beginner workout plans and join their forums to connect with like-minded individuals.

Precision Nutrition

Description: Precision Nutrition offers educational resources on nutrition and fitness, as well as personalized coaching programs.

Trending Insight: The website's focus on science-based information and practical application makes it a valuable resource. **Example:** Explore Precision Nutrition's articles on macronutrients, meal planning, and exercise to enhance your understanding and approach to weight loss.

Courses

Coursera: "The Science of Well-Being" by Yale University

Description: This popular online course explores the science behind happiness and well-being, offering strategies to improve mental and emotional health.

Trending Insight: Understanding the connection between mental health and weight management can help create a holistic approach to your journey.

Example: Apply the course's techniques for increasing happiness and reducing stress to support your weight loss efforts.

Udemy: "Fitness Nutrition Certification"

Description: This course covers the fundamentals of nutrition, diet planning, and weight management, providing a comprehensive understanding of how to fuel your body.

Trending Insight: Gaining a deeper knowledge of nutrition can empower you to make informed choices and create effective meal plans. **Example:** Use the knowledge from the course to design a balanced and sustainable diet that supports your weight loss goals.

CONCLUSION

Hey Fella, Time to Lose Weight

As we come to the end of "Hey Fella, Time to Lose Weight," it's time to reflect on the journey we've embarked upon together and the roadmap we've laid out for a healthier, happier, and more vibrant life. This book is more than just a guide to shedding pounds; it's a comprehensive toolkit designed to empower you to take control of your health, transform your lifestyle, and sustain these changes for the long term.

Embracing the Journey

Weight loss is not merely about numbers on a scale; it's about reclaiming your life and harnessing the energy and confidence to live it to the fullest. As we've explored, a successful weight loss journey is built on several pillars: the right mindset, proper nutrition, effective exercise, sustainable lifestyle changes, ongoing motivation, and robust support systems. By integrating these elements into your daily routine, you set yourself up for lasting success.

The Right Mindset: Preparing for Success

We started by emphasizing the importance of a positive and realistic mindset. Setting attainable goals, maintaining a positive attitude, and overcoming common obstacles are foundational to any weight loss journey. Current trends emphasize the psychological aspects of weight management, including mindfulness and self-compassion, which help in creating a sustainable and enjoyable path to health.

Proper Nutrition: Fueling Your Body Right

Understanding the role of calories and macronutrients, planning simple and nutritious meals, and adopting smart snacking habits are key to effective weight loss. With the help of technology and modern trends, such as the Mediterranean diet or intermittent fasting, we can navigate our dietary choices more effectively. We've learned how to use apps to track our intake, understand our food better, and make healthier choices consistently.

Effective Exercise: Moving Toward a Healthier You

Finding the right workout, incorporating physical activity into your day, and balancing home workouts with gym routines were explored to make exercise a sustainable part of your lifestyle. The rise of online fitness communities and streaming workouts has made it easier than ever to stay active, no matter your schedule or location. If you make exercise fun and mix it up, you'll probably keep at it.

Sustainable Lifestyle Changes: Small Tweaks, Big Results

Small but consistent changes can lead to significant results. Adequate sleep, stress management, and building healthy habits are critical components that often go overlooked. The interconnectedness of these factors with weight management was highlighted, showing how improving one aspect of your life can positively influence others.

Ongoing Motivation: Keeping the Momentum Going

Staying motivated is a challenge many face. By tracking progress, celebrating milestones, and drawing inspiration from success stories, we can keep our spirits high. Social media, fitness apps, and wearable technology play significant roles in keeping us motivated and accountable.

Robust Support Systems: Tools and Support for Your Journey

Leveraging resources like recommended apps and websites, joining community and support groups, and continually learning through books and courses can provide the necessary support and knowledge. Engaging with others on similar journeys fosters a sense of community and provides invaluable encouragement and advice.

As we come to the end of "Hey Fella, Time to Lose Weight," it's time to reflect on the journey we've embarked upon together and the roadmap we've laid out for a healthier, happier, and more vibrant life. This book is more than just a guide to shedding pounds; it's a comprehensive toolkit designed to empower you to take control of your health, transform your lifestyle, and sustain these changes for the long term.

Finding the right workout, incorporating physical activity into your day, and balancing home workouts with gym routines were explored to make exercise a sustainable part of your lifestyle. The rise of online fitness communities and streaming workouts has made it easier than ever to stay active, no matter your schedule or location. When you make exercise interesting and diverse, you're more apt to continue doing it. Sustainable Lifestyle Changes: Small Tweaks, Big Results

Small but consistent changes can lead to significant results. Adequate sleep, stress management, and building healthy habits are critical components that often go overlooked. The interconnectedness of these factors with weight management was highlighted, showing how improving one aspect of your life can positively influence others.

Beyond the Scale

A recurring theme throughout this book is that weight loss should be about improving overall health and well-being rather than merely hitting a target weight. There are benefits to be gained from this journey that go beyond what can be measured on the scale:

Increased Energy Levels: Shedding excess weight and eating a balanced diet can lead to higher energy levels, allowing you to engage more fully in daily activities and pursue your passions.

Improved Mental Health: Regular exercise, a nutritious diet, and adequate sleep contribute significantly to better mental health. You'll likely find yourself feeling happier, less stressed, and more focused.

Enhanced Self-Confidence: As you make progress and achieve your goals, your self-confidence will grow. This newfound confidence can have a positive impact on all areas of your life, from personal relationships to professional endeavors.

Long-Term Health Benefits: Maintaining a healthy weight reduces the risk of chronic diseases such as diabetes, heart disease, and certain cancers. Investing in your health now pays dividends in the form of a longer, healthier life.

The Power of Community

One of the most powerful tools in your weight loss arsenal is the support of others. The presence of a support network, be it from family, friends, or online communities, can truly make a difference. Sharing your journey, celebrating successes, and leaning on others during challenging times can provide the motivation and encouragement you need to keep going.

Adapting and Evolving

It's essential to remember that your weight loss journey is not static. As you progress, your goals and needs may evolve. Regularly revisiting your plans, adjusting your strategies, and setting new challenges can keep your journey dynamic and engaging. Whether it's training for a new physical challenge, trying a different dietary approach, or finding new ways to stay active, adaptability is key.

Final Thoughts

"Hey Fella, Time to Lose Weight" is not just a book; it's a companion on your journey to better health. The principles and strategies outlined here are designed to be practical, sustainable, and empowering. Remember, the journey to weight loss and better health is personal, and there is no one-size-fits-all approach. What matters most is finding what works for you and staying committed to your goals.

Your journey is unique, and it's important to honor and respect your path. Embrace the good and the bad, take lessons from every moment, and always move forward. With the right mindset, tools, and support, you can achieve and maintain your weight loss goals, leading to a healthier, happier, and more fulfilling life. Thank you for allowing this book to be a part of your journey, and here's to your continued success and well-being!

END

www.ingramcontent.com/pod-product-compliance
Lightning Source LLC
Chambersburg PA
CBHW081448250726
48662CB00009B/2988